HOW TO GET

DREADLOCKS

A Comprehensive Step-by-Step Guide
to Starting, Styling, and Maintaining
Your Locs

Gerald S. Milligan

ALL RIGHT RESERVED @ 2024

Gerald S. Milligan

CONTENTS

Preface

T his book is a result of my personal love and curiosity for dreadlocks, and my desire to share my knowledge and experience with others who are interested in this unique and fascinating hairstyle. I have been wearing dreadlocks over the years, and I have learned a lot about the history, culture, and art of dreadlocks, as well as the practical parts of starting, styling, and maintaining dreadlocks.

In this book, I have tried to provide a complete and informative guide to dreadlocks, that covers everything from the basics to the advanced topics, and that caters to different hair types, textures, lengths, and preferences. I have also tried to make this book fun and engaging, by including some personal stories, tips, tricks, and pictures, that show the diversity and beauty of dreadlocks, and the people who wear them.

My goal with this book is to inspire and teach anyone who wants to learn more about dreadlocks, whether they are new to dreadlocks, or they have been rocking them for years. I also hope that this book will help you respect and embrace your dreadlocks, and to express your individuality and creativity through them.

Forward

Dreadlocks are more than just a haircut. They are a way of life, a symbol of personality, and a form of art. Dreadlocks have a long and rich past that spans across different cultures, religions, and regions of the world. Dreadlocks have also been linked with different meanings and values, such as spirituality, resistance, freedom, and beauty.

In this book, you will find a full guide to dreadlocks, that will teach you everything you need to know about dreadlocks, from how to start them, to how to style them, to how to maintain them. You will also find some of the benefits and difficulties of having dreadlocks, as well as some of the myths and misconceptions that surround them.

This book is written by a fellow dreadlock lover and enthusiast, who has been wearing dreadlocks for over 10 years, and who has learned a lot from his own experience and study. He has also included some personal stories, tips, tricks, and pictures, that will make this book more interesting and fun.

Whether you are new to dreadlocks, or you have been rocking them for years, this book will help you learn more about this unique and interesting hairstyle. This book will also inspire you to embrace and enjoy your dreadlocks, and to show your individuality and creativity through them.

I highly suggest this book to anyone who wants to get dreadlocks, or who wants to improve their dreadlocks, or who simply wants to appreciate and understand dreadlocks. This book is a must-have for any dreadlock lover and fan.

Chapter One

How to Start Dreadlocks

If you have chosen to get dreadlocks, you may be wondering how to start them. There are many different methods and techniques that you can use to start your dreadlocks, based on your hair type, texture, length, and desired look. In this chapter, we will explain some of the most common and popular ways for starting dreadlocks, and how to use them. We will also tell you what tools and goods you need to start your dreadlocks, and where to get them.

Choosing the Right Method for Your Hair Type and Desired Look

Before you start your dreadlocks, you need to choose the right way for your hair type and desired look. Different ways work better for different hair types and textures, and they also create different effects and results. Here are some of the factors that you need to consider when picking the right method for your hair type and desired look:

- **Your hair type**: Your hair type refers to the thickness, texture, and curl pattern of your hair. Generally, there are four main hair types: straight, wavy, curly, and kinky. Each hair type has its own benefits and disadvantages when it comes to starting dreadlocks. For example, straight hair tends to be more slippery and less prone to tangling, which makes it harder to start dreadlocks, but easier to keep them. On the other hand, kinky hair tends to be coarser and frizzier, which makes it easier to start dreadlocks, but harder to keep them.

- **Your hair texture**: Your hair texture refers to the diameter, porosity, and flexibility of your hair strands. Generally, there are three main hair textures: fine, medium, and coarse. Each hair texture has its own characteristics and difficulties when it comes to starting dreadlocks. For example, fine hair tends to be softer and silkier, which makes it more difficult to start dreadlocks, but more controllable and flexible. On the other hand, coarse hair tends to be rougher and stiffer, which makes it easier to start dreadlocks, but more rigid and brittle.

- **Your hair length**: Your hair length refers to how long your hair is, from the roots to the tips. Generally, there are three main hair lengths: short, medium, and long. Each hair length has its own requirements and limits when it comes to starting dreadlocks. For example, short hair tends to be more convenient and comfortable, but it may not have enough length to make dreadlocks, or to create different styles. On the other hand, long hair tends to be more versatile and expressive, but it may be heavier and more cumbersome, or take longer to make dreadlocks.

- **Your chosen look**: Your preferred look refers to how you want your dreadlocks to look, in terms of size, shape, and style. Generally, there are three main types of dreadlocks: thin, medium, and thick. Each type of dreadlocks has its own pros and cons when it comes to starting dreadlocks. For example, thin dreadlocks tend to be neater and cleaner, but they may also be more fragile and prone to breaking. On the other hand, thick dreadlocks tend to be stronger and more lasting, but they may also be more bulky and unruly.

Based on these factors, you can choose the method that suits your hair type and intended look the best. next We'll discuss some of the most common and popular ways for starting dreadlocks, and how they work

The Backcombing Method for Fine or Straight Hair

The backcombing method is one of the most widely used and successful methods for starting dreadlocks, especially for fine or straight hair. It involves using a fine-toothed comb to tease and tangle your hair into pieces, and then rolling and twisting them into dreadlocks. This method produces tight and uniform dreadlocks, that can last for a long time. However, this method can also be time-consuming and painful, and it can damage your hair and scalp if done wrong. Here are the steps to take when using the backcombing method:

- Wash and dry your hair fully, and avoid using any conditioner or product that can make your hair slippery or oily.

- Divide your hair into equal parts, depending on how thick or thin you want your dreadlocks to be. You can use rubber bands, clips, or pins to hold the pieces in place.

- Take one piece of hair, and comb it from the tips to the roots, using a fine-toothed comb. This will create knots and kinks in your hair, and form a matted base for your dreadlock. You may need to repeat this process several times, until your hair is fully backcombed.

- Roll and twist the backcombed section of hair between your hands, in a clockwise or counterclockwise direction. This will tighten and smooth out your dreadlock, and give it a cylindrical shape. You may need to add some gel or wax to hold your dreadlock in place.

- Repeat the same process with the rest of the parts of hair, until you have formed all your dreadlocks.

- Secure the tips of your dreadlocks with rubber bands, beads, or rings, to keep them from unraveling.

The Twisting Method for Thick or Curly Hair

The twisting method is another famous and effective method for starting dreadlocks, especially for thick or curly hair. It includes using your fingers or a comb to twist your hair into sections, and then rolling and twisting them into dreadlocks. This method makes loose and natural dreadlocks, that can grow and mature over time. However, this way can also be less stable and durable, and it can require more maintenance and care. Here are the steps to follow when using the turning method:

- Wash and condition your hair thoroughly, and towel-dry it until it is damp but not wet.
- Divide your hair into equal parts, depending on how thick or thin you want your dreadlocks to be. You can use rubber bands, clips, or pins to hold the pieces in place.
- Take one piece of hair, and twist it from the roots to the tips, using your fingers or a comb. This will make a spiral or coil in your hair, and form a loose base for your dreadlock. You may need to add some gel or wax to hold your twist in place.
- Roll and twist the twisted section of hair between your palms, in the same way as your twist. This will tighten and smooth out your dreadlock, and give it a cylindrical shape. You may need to add some more gel or wax to hold your dreadlock in place.

- Repeat the same process with the rest of the parts of hair, until you have formed all your dreadlocks.
- Secure the tips of your dreadlocks with rubber bands, beads, or rings, to prevent them from breaking.

The Neglect Method for Natural and Freeform Dreadlocks

The neglect method is the most natural and organic method for starting dreadlocks, as it includes letting your hair form dreadlocks on its own, without any interference or manipulation. It works best for kinky or wavy hair, as it tends to lock up faster and easier than other hair types. This method produces unique and freeform dreadlocks, that can vary in size, shape, and style. However, this method can also be unpredictable and uncontrollable, and it can take a long time to make dreadlocks. Here are the steps to follow when using the ignoring method:

- Wash and dry your hair fully, and avoid using any conditioner or product that can prevent your hair from locking up.
- Stop combing, brushing, or detangling your hair, and let it form knots and kinks naturally. You can use your fingers to separate your hair into parts, or let it form sections on its own.
- Let your hair grow and mature, and watch it form dreadlocks over time. This can take anywhere from a few months to a few years, based on your hair type, length, and growth rate.
- Wash your hair occasionally, but not too often, and use a residue-free shampoo that can keep your hair clean and healthy. You can also use a spray or a rinse to moisturize your hair and scalp, and to avoid dryness and itchiness.

- Maintain your dreadlocks by hand rolling them occasionally, or by using a crochet hook or a needle to tighten and repair them. You can also shape or cut your dreadlocks if they become too long or uneven.

The Tools and Products You Need to Start Your Dreadlocks

To start your dreadlocks, you will need some tools and products that can help you create and keep your dreadlocks. Here are some of the tools and goods that you will need, and where to get them:

- **A fine-toothed comb**: A fine-toothed comb is a tool that you can use to backcomb your hair into dreadlocks. It can make tight and uniform dreadlocks, and it can work for any hair type or texture. You can get a fine-toothed comb from any beauty supply shop, or online.

- **A crochet hook or a needle**: A crochet hook or a needle is a tool that you can use to fix and repair your dreadlocks. It can help you fix any loose hairs or gaps in your dreadlocks, and make them neater and more regular. You can get a crochet hook or a needle from any craft shop, or online.

- **A gel or a wax**: A gel or a wax is a product that you can use to hold your dreadlocks in place, and to prevent them from breaking or frizzing. It can also help you shape and style your dreadlocks, and give them some shine and wetness. You should use a gel or a wax that is carefully formulated for dreadlocks, or a natural alternative, such as honey, beeswax, or flaxseed gel. You can get a gel or a wax from any beauty supply shop, or online.

- **A shampoo**: A shampoo is a product that you can use to wash your dreadlocks, and to keep them clean and healthy. It can also help you clear any dirt, oil, or residue from your scalp and hair, and to avoid odors and infections. You should use a shampoo that is residue-free, soft, and pH-balanced, and that does not contain any sulfates, parabens, or silicones. You can get a shampoo from any beauty supply shop, or online.

- **A conditioner**: A conditioner is a product that you can use to condition your dreadlocks, and to keep them soft and moist. It can also help you detangle and moisturize your dreadlocks, and to avoid dryness and breakage. You should use a conditioner that is lightweight, water-based, and oil-free, and that does not contain any sulfates, chemicals, or silicones. You can get a conditioner from any beauty supply shop, or online.

- **An oil or a moisturizer**: An oil or a moisturizer is a product that you can use to oil or moisturize your dreadlocks, and to keep them healthy and wet. It can also help you seal in the moisture and nutrients in your dreadlocks, and to avoid dryness and dullness. You should use an oil or a moisturizer that is natural, organic, and clean, and that does not contain any mineral oil, petroleum, or alcohol. You can get an oil or a moisturizer from any health food shop, or online.

Chapter Two

How to Style Dreadlocks

Once you have started your dreadlocks, you may want to try with different styles and looks. Styling your dreadlocks can be fun and creative, and it can also help you show your personality and mood. In this part, we will show you some of the basic techniques for styling your dreadlocks, as well as some of the different types of dreadlock styles and how to achieve them. We will also give you some tips on the accessories and embellishments you can use to improve your dreadlocks, and how to keep your dreadlocks neat and tidy.

Basic Techniques for Styling Your Dreadlocks

There are some basic methods that you can use to style your dreadlocks, regardless of their length, thickness, or texture. These methods include:

- **Tying**: You can use elastic bands, hair ties, or clips to tie your dreadlocks into a ponytail, a bun, a half-up, or any other way you like. Tying your dreadlocks can help you keep them out of your face, or create a more official or casual look. You can also tie some of your dreadlocks together to make sections or patterns.

- **Braiding**: You can braid your dreadlocks together to make different shapes and textures. You can braid your dreadlocks into one big braid, or several smaller braids. You can also braid your dreadlocks with other materials, such as ribbons, beads, or yarn, to add some color and variety. Braiding your dreadlocks can help you create a more detailed or elegant look, or a more playful or funky look.

- **Twisting**: You can twist your dreadlocks together to make coils, curls, or waves. You can twist your dreadlocks into one big twist, or several smaller twists. You can also twist your dreadlocks with other materials, such as wire, string, or rubber bands, to create different forms and effects. Twisting your dreadlocks can help you create a more natural or organic look, or a more edgy or artistic look.

- **Pinning**: You can use pins, clips, or combs to pin your dreadlocks into different places or directions. You can pin your dreadlocks up, down, sideways, or diagonally. You can also pin your dreadlocks into different forms, such as a mohawk, a faux hawk, or a crown. Pinning your dreadlocks can help you create a more dramatic or bold look, or a more subtle or polished look.

Different Types of Dreadlock Styles and How to Achieve Them

There are many different types of dreadlock styles that you can try, based on your preference, occasion, and mood. Some of the most famous and common dreadlock styles are:

- **The Classic:** This is the easiest and most versatile dreadlock style. It includes leaving your dreadlocks loose and free, and letting them fall naturally. This style works well for any length, thickness, or texture of dreadlocks, and it can fit any face shape or personality. To achieve this look, you just need to wash and dry your dreadlocks regularly, and separate them if they start to stick together. You can also add some accessories or ornaments to spice up this style, such as beads, rings, or feathers.

- **The Updo:** This is a more elegant and sophisticated dreadlock look. It includes tying your dreadlocks into a bun, a knot, or a chignon, and securing them with pins, clips, or bands. This style works well for medium to long dreadlocks, and it can create a more polished or business look. To achieve this look, you need to gather your dreadlocks at the top, back, or side of your head, and twist them into a bun, a knot, or a chignon. You can also leave some dreadlocks loose or braided to frame your face, or add some accessories or embellishments to improve this style, such as flowers, pearls, or crystals.

- **The Ponytail**: This is a more casual and sportier dreadlock look. It includes tying your dreadlocks into a ponytail, and letting them hang down your back or over your shoulder. This style works well for any length, thickness, or roughness.

- **The Braid-Out**: This is a more textured and voluminous dreadlock look. It includes braiding your dreadlocks into several smaller braids, and then taking them out after a few hours or overnight. This style works well for any length, thickness, or texture of dreadlocks, and it can give a more curly or wavy look. To achieve this look, you need to wash and condition your dreadlocks, and then braid them into several smaller braids while they are still damp. You can also add some gel or wax to keep the braids in place. Then, you need to let your dreadlocks dry completely, either by air-drying or using a heater. Once they are dry, you can take out the knots and fluff your dreadlocks with your fingers.

You can also add some oil or spray to give your dreadlocks some shine and wetness.

- **The High-Top**: This is a more modern and trendier dreadlock look. It includes shaving the sides and back of your head, and leaving your dreadlocks on the top of your head. This style works well for short to medium dreadlocks, and it can create a more edgy or funky look. To achieve this style, you need to visit a barber or a designer who can shave the sides and back of your head, and shape your dreadlocks on the top of your head. You can also ask them to remove or taper the shaved areas, or to create some designs or patterns with the razor. You can also style your dreadlocks on the top of your head in different ways, such as putting them into a bun, a ponytail, or a mohawk.

- **The Criss-Cross**: This is a more complex and elaborate dreadlock style. It includes crossing your dreadlocks over each other, and pinning them into different positions or directions. This style works well for medium to long dreadlocks, and it can create a more artistic or mature look. To achieve this style, you need to have some pins, clips, or combs ready. Then, you need to take two dreadlocks from opposite sides of your head, and cross them over each other. You can then pin them into place, either at the back, the top, or the side of your head. You can repeat this process with more dreadlocks, until you have made a crisscross pattern all over your head. You can also leave some dreadlocks loose or braided to frame your face, or to add some contrast to the crisscross design.

Accessories and Embellishments for Your Dreadlocks

One of the fun and artistic aspects of having dreadlocks is that you can accessorize and embellish them in various ways. You can use different materials, colors, and shapes to enhance your dreadlocks, and to show your personality and mood. Some of the decorations and embellishments that you can use for your dreadlocks are:

- **Beads**: Beads are one of the most common and popular decorations for dreadlocks. They come in different sizes, shapes, colors, and materials, such as wood, metal, glass, or plastic. You can use beads to decorate your dreadlocks, or to keep them in place. You can also use beads to make different patterns or designs on your dreadlocks, such as stripes, dots, or spirals. To use beads, you just need to slide them onto your dreadlocks, and fix them with a knot or a rubber band. You can also use a crochet hook or a needle to help you place the beads onto your dreadlocks.

- **Rings**: Rings are another common and popular ornament for dreadlocks. They are similar to beads, but they are usually made of metal, such as silver, gold, or copper. You can use rings to adorn your dreadlocks, or to join them together. You can also use rings to make different shapes or effects on your dreadlocks, such as loops, twists, or chains. To use rings, you just need to open them slightly, and then close them around your dreadlocks. You can also use a plier or a tweezer to help you fix the rings on your dreadlocks.

- **Feathers**: Feathers are a more natural and organic decoration for dreadlocks. They come in different colors, sizes, and types, such as peacock, ostrich, or parrot. You can use feathers to add some flair and color to your dreadlocks, or to create a more artistic or tribal look. To use feathers, you just need to connect them to your dreadlocks with some thread, wire, or glue. You can also use a bead or a ring to bind the feathers to your dreadlocks.

- **Ribbons**: Ribbons are a more feminine and romantic decoration for dreadlocks. They come in different colors, designs, and materials, such as silk, cotton, or lace. You can use ribbons to wrap around your dreadlocks, or to tie them into bows or knots. You can also use ribbons to create different styles or looks on your dreadlocks, such as bands, twists, or curls. To use ribbons, you just need to cut them into the desired length, and then wrap or tie them around your dreadlocks. You can also use a pin or a clip to hold the ribbons in place on your dreadlocks.

Tips and Tricks for Keeping Your Dreadlocks Neat and Tidy

While dreadlocks are a low-maintenance haircut, they still require some care and attention to keep them neat and tidy. Here are some tips and tricks that you can follow to keep your dreadlocks looking their best:

- Wash your dreadlocks regularly, but not too often. Washing your dreadlocks helps to clear dirt, oil, and residue from your scalp and hair, and to avoid odors and infections. However, washing your dreadlocks too often can dry out your hair and skin, and loosen your dreadlocks. The ideal frequency of washing your dreadlocks depends on your hair type, texture, and lifestyle, but usually, once or twice a week is enough. You should also use a mild shampoo that is carefully formulated for dreadlocks, or a natural alternative, such as baking soda, apple cider vinegar, or lemon juice. You should also rinse your dreadlocks fully, and squeeze out the excess water.

- Dry your dreadlocks properly, and avoid using heat. Drying your dreadlocks properly helps to prevent mold, mildew, and bacteria from growing in your hair, and to keep the shape and integrity of your dreadlocks. However, using heat to dry your dreadlocks can damage your hair and skin, and cause your dreadlocks to become brittle and frizzy. The best way to dry your dreadlocks is to let them air-dry, or to use a microfiber towel or a cotton t-shirt to gently blot them. You can also use a dryer on a low or cool setting, but only for a few minutes, and at a safe distance from your head and hair.

- Moisturize your dreadlocks regularly, but not too much. Moisturizing your dreadlocks helps to keep your hair and head healthy and hydrated, and to prevent your dreadlocks from becoming dry and dull. However, moisturizing your dreadlocks too much can make your hair and head greasy and oily, and attract dirt and dust to your dreadlocks. The ideal amount of moisturizing your dreadlocks depends on your hair type, texture, and climate, but usually, once or twice a week is enough. You should also use a natural oil or a moisturizer that is specially designed for dreadlocks, or a homemade mixture, such as aloe vera gel, coconut oil, or shea butter. You should also apply the oil or moisturizer lightly, and massage it into your scalp and hair.

- Separate your dreadlocks regularly, and avoid joining them. Separating your dreadlocks regularly helps to prevent them from growing together, and to keep the size and shape of your dreadlocks. However, combining your dreadlocks can make them thicker and heavier, and cause tightness and stress on your scalp and hair. The ideal frequency of separating your dreadlocks depends on how fast your hair grows, and how tight your dreadlocks are, but usually, once or twice a week is enough.

Chapter Three

How to Maintain Dreadlocks

Having dreadlocks is not a one-time thing. It is a continuous process that needs regular maintenance and care. Maintaining your dreadlocks can help you keep them healthy, beautiful, and strong, and prevent them from becoming messy, broken, or infected. In this chapter, we will show you some of the best practices for washing and drying your dreadlocks, as well as some of the essential oils and moisturizers for keeping your dreadlocks hydrated and fed. We will also teach you some of the crochet hook and palm rolling methods for tightening and repairing your dreadlocks, and some of the answers for common dreadlock problems and issues.

The Best Practices for Washing and Drying Your Dreadlocks

Washing and drying your dreadlocks are two of the most important aspects of keeping your dreadlocks, as they can affect the cleanliness, health, and appearance of your dreadlocks. Here are some of the best techniques for washing and drying your dreadlocks:

- Wash your dreadlocks regularly, but not too often. Washing your dreadlocks helps to clear dirt, oil, and residue from your scalp and hair, and to avoid odors and infections. However, washing your dreadlocks too often can dry out your hair and skin, and loosen your dreadlocks. The ideal frequency of washing your dreadlocks depends on your hair type, texture, and lifestyle, but usually, once or twice a week is enough. You should also use a mild shampoo that is carefully formulated for dreadlocks, or a natural alternative, such as baking soda, apple cider vinegar, or lemon juice. You should also rinse your dreadlocks carefully, and squeeze out the excess water.

- Dry your dreadlocks properly, and avoid using heat. Drying your dreadlocks properly helps to prevent mold, mildew, and bacteria from growing in your hair, and to keep the shape and integrity of your dreadlocks. However, using heat to dry your dreadlocks can damage your hair and skin, and cause your dreadlocks to become brittle and frizzy. The best way to dry your dreadlocks is to let them air-dry, or to use a microfiber towel or a cotton t-shirt to gently blot them. You can also use a dryer on a low or cool setting, but only for a few minutes, and at a safe distance from your head and hair.

The Essential Oils and Moisturizers for Keeping Your Dreadlocks Hydrated and Nourished

Oiling and moisturizing your dreadlocks are two of the most important aspects of maintaining your dreadlocks, as they can affect the health, hydration, and nourishment of your dreadlocks. Here are some of the key oils and moisturizers for keeping your dreadlocks hydrated and nourished:

- **Coconut oil:** Coconut oil is one of the most famous and beneficial oils for dreadlocks, as it can penetrate deep into your hair and scalp, and provide them with moisture, nutrients, and protection. Coconut oil can also help you avoid dryness, dullness, and breakage, and give your dreadlocks a soft and shiny look. You can use coconut oil as a pre-wash treatment, by applying it to your scalp and hair, and letting it for 15 to 30 minutes before washing. You can also use coconut oil as a post-wash treatment, by applying a small amount to your damp or dry dreadlocks, and massaging it into your head and hair.

- **Aloe vera gel**: Aloe vera gel is another popular and beneficial moisturizer for dreadlocks, as it can soothe and heal your skin and hair, and provide them with hydration, vitamins, and minerals. Aloe vera gel can also help you avoid itchiness, inflammation, and dandruff, and give your dreadlocks a smooth and silky look. You can use aloe vera gel as a leave-in conditioner, by applying it to your damp or dry dreadlocks, and spreading it evenly throughout your head and hair. You can also use aloe vera gel as a spray, by mixing it with some water, and spraying it onto your dreadlocks whenever they feel dry or curly.

The Crochet Hook and Palm Rolling Methods for Tightening and Repairing Your Dreadlocks

Tightening and repairing your dreadlocks are two of the most common and useful aspects of keeping your dreadlocks, as they can affect the stability, durability, and appearance of your dreadlocks. Here are some of the crochet hook and palm rolling ways for tightening and repairing your dreadlocks:

- **The crochet hook method**: The crochet hook method is a method that you can use to tighten and repair your dreadlocks, by using a crochet hook to pull and weave any free hairs or gaps into your dreadlocks. This method can help you make your dreadlocks neater and more regular, and fix any flaws or mistakes in your dreadlocks. To use the crochet hook method, you need to have a crochet hook that is small enough to fit into your dreadlocks, and that has a smooth and rounded tip. You also need to have some time and skill, as this method can be tricky and tedious. Here are the steps to take when using the crochet hook method:

- Wash and dry your dreadlocks carefully, and avoid using any conditioner or product that can make your hair slippery or oily.
- Take one dreadlock, and check it for any loose hairs or gaps. You can also use your fingers to feel for any bumps or lumps in your dreadlock.
- Insert the crochet hook into your dreadlock, near the loose hair or gap, and hook the free hair with the tip of the crochet hook. You can also use the crochet hook to pick up some hair from the dreadlock, and make a loop.
- Pull the crochet hook out of the dreadlock, and bring the loose hair or loop into the dreadlock. You can also

use the crochet hook to tuck the loose hair or loop into the dreadlock, and make it more secure.

- Repeat the same process with the rest of the loose hairs or gaps in your dreadlock, until you have tightened and corrected your dreadlock.
- Repeat the same process with the rest of your dreadlocks, until you have tightened and fixed all your dreadlocks.

- **The palm rolling method**: The palm rolling method is a method that you can use to tighten and smooth your dreadlocks, by rolling them between your hands, in a clockwise or counterclockwise direction. This method can help you compress and shape your dreadlocks, and give them a cylindrical and regular look. To use the hand rolling method, you need to have some gel or wax that can hold your dreadlocks in place, and that can provide some friction and resistance.

You also need to have some time and energy, as this method can be repetitive and tiring. Here are the steps to follow when using the palm rolling method:

- Wash and dry your dreadlocks thoroughly, and add some gel or wax to your dreadlocks, sparingly and evenly.
- Take one dreadlock, and place it between your hands, near the roots. You can also use your fingers to remove your dreadlock from the others, and to hold it in place.
- Roll your dreadlock between your palms, in a clockwise or counterclockwise direction, based on your preference. You can also add some pressure and speed to your rolling, depending on how tight or smooth you want your dreadlock to be.
- Move your palms along your dreadlock, from the roots to the tips,

and roll your dreadlock between your palms, until you have strengthened and smoothed your dreadlock.

- Repeat the same process with the rest of your dreadlocks, until you have tightened and smoothed all your dreadlocks.

The Solutions for Common Dreadlock Problems and Issues

Having dreadlocks can also come with some problems and issues, that can affect the health, comfort, and look of your dreadlocks. Here are some of the common dreadlock problems and issues, and some of the answers for them:

- **Frizz**: Frizz is a problem that happens when your dreadlocks become fuzzy, flyaway, or unruly, due to humidity, dryness, or damage. Frizz can make your dreadlocks look messy and unattractive, and it can also cause your dreadlocks to lose their shape and structure. To avoid or reduce frizz, you can:

- Use a satin or silk pillowcase, scarf, or bonnet, to protect your dreadlocks from friction and static, when you sleep or journey.
- Use a spray or a rinse, made of water and aloe vera gel, rose water, or lavender oil, to hydrate and smooth your dreadlocks, whenever they feel dry or curly.
- Use a crochet hook or a needle, to tuck any loose hairs or frizz into your dreadlocks, and make them neater and tidier.

- **Lint**: Lint is a problem that happens when your dreadlocks collect small pieces of fabric, dust, or dirt, from your clothing, bedding, or environment. Lint can make your dreadlocks look dirty and dull, and it can also cause your dreadlocks to become heavy and stiff. To avoid or remove lint, you can:

- Use a lint roller, a sticky tape, or a tweezers, to pick out any obvious lint from your dreadlocks, and make them cleaner and shinier.
- Use a dark-colored or lint-free clothing, bedding, or towel, to avoid spreading any lint to your dreadlocks, and make them more lint-free and vibrant.
- Use a clarifying shampoo or a vinegar rinse, to wash your dreadlocks once in a while, and clear any build-up or residue from your dreadlocks, and make them fresher and lighter.

- **Itchiness**: Itchiness is a problem that happens when your scalp becomes irritated, inflamed, or infected, due to dryness, dirt, or germs. Itchiness can make your dreadlocks uncomfortable and unpleasant, and it can also cause you to scratch your head and damage your dreadlocks. To avoid or relieve itchiness, you can:

- Use a spray or a rinse, made of water and tea tree oil, peppermint oil, or lavender oil, to soothe and heal your scalp, and avoid itchiness and infection.
- Use a shampoo or a conditioner, that includes soothing and moisturizing ingredients, such as aloe vera, oatmeal, or chamomile, to hydrate and nourish your scalp, and prevent dryness and inflammation.
- Use a scalp massager or a brush, to gently massage your head and stimulate blood circulation, and relieve itchiness and tension.

- **Dandruff**: Dandruff is a problem that appears when your scalp produces excess flakes of dead skin, due to dryness, oiliness, or fungus. Dandruff can make your dreadlocks look flaky and dirty, and it can also cause your head to itch and smell. To avoid or reduce dandruff, you can:

- Use a shampoo or a rinse, that includes anti-dandruff and anti-fungal ingredients, such as zinc pyrithione, selenium sulfide, or apple cider vinegar, to cleanse and balance your scalp, and prevent dandruff and fungus.
- Use a spray or a rinse, made of water and lemon juice, rosemary oil, or thyme oil, to refresh and tone your scalp, and avoid dandruff and odor.
- Use a scalp exfoliator or a scrub, made of sugar, salt, or baking soda, to gently remove any dead skin or flakes from your head, and prevent dandruff and build-up.

Conclusion

You have reached the end of this book, and we hope that you have learned a lot about dreadlocks, from how to start them, to how to style them, to how to keep them. We also hope that you have loved and appreciated the diversity and beauty of dreadlocks, and the people who wear them.

Dreadlocks are more than just a haircut. They are a statement, a lifestyle, and a community. Dreadlocks can help you show your individuality and creativity, and connect with your spirituality and heritage. Dreadlocks can also push you to overcome stereotypes and prejudices, and to embrace your natural and authentic self.

We encourage you to continue your journey with dreadlocks, and to explore the different methods, techniques, styles, and accessories that you can use to make and enhance your dreadlocks. We also welcome you to share your experiences and feedback with us, and to join the online and offline communities of dreadlock lovers and enthusiasts.

Thank you for reading this book, and for deciding to get dreadlocks. We wish you all the best, and we hope that you will love and enjoy your dreadlocks as much as we do.